HOW TO TREAT AND MANAGE SHOULDER PAIN

Rantho Mahlare MD

CONTENT

SHOULDER PAIN

Overview

Physical uneasiness of the shoulder, including the joint itself or the muscles, ligaments and tendons that help the joint.

The shoulder has a wide and adaptable scope of movement. When something turns out badly with your shoulder, it hampers your capacity to move unreservedly and can cause a lot of torment and distress.

The shoulder is a ball-and-attachment joint that has three primary bones: the humerus (long arm bone), the clavicle (collarbone), and the scapula (otherwise called the shoulder bone).

These bones are padded by a layer of ligament. There are two principle joints. The acromioclavicular joint is between the most noteworthy aspect of the scapula and the clavicle.

The glenohumeral joint is comprised of the top, ball-formed aspect of the humerus bone and the external edge of the scapula. This joint is otherwise called the shoulder joint.

The shoulder joint is the most versatile joint in the body. It pushes the shoulder ahead and in reverse. It likewise permits the arm to move in a roundabout movement and to go far up into the clouds from the body.

Shoulders get their scope of movement from the rotator sleeve.

The rotator sleeve is comprised of four ligaments. Ligaments are the tissues that interface muscles to bone. It might be excruciating or hard to lift your arm over your head if the ligaments or bones around the rotator sleeve are harmed or swollen.

You can harm your shoulder by performing physical work, playing sports, or even by monotonous development. Certain sicknesses can achieve torment that movements to the shoulder. These incorporate illnesses of the cervical spine (neck), just as liver, heart, or gallbladder sickness.

You're bound to have issues with your shoulder as you become more established, particularly after age 60. This is on the grounds that the delicate tissues encompassing the shoulder will in general deteriorate with age.

As a rule, you can treat shoulder torment at home. Nonetheless, exercise-based recuperation, meds, or medical procedure may likewise be fundamental.

This is what you need think about shoulder torment, including causes, analysis, treatment, and anticipation.

What causes shoulder torment?

A few factors and conditions can add to bear torment. The most pervasive reason is rotator sleeve tendinitis.

This is a condition described by swollen ligaments. Another regular reason for shoulder torment is impingement disorder where the rotator sleeve gets captured between the acromium (part of the scapula that covers the ball) and humeral head (the ball bit of the humerus).

In some cases, shoulder torment is the consequence of injury to another area in your body, ordinarily the neck or biceps. This is known as alluded torment. Alluded torment for the most part doesn't deteriorate when you move your shoulder.

Different reasons for shoulder torment include:

- joint inflammation
- torn ligament

- torn rotator sleeve

- swollen bursa sacs or ligaments

- bone prods (hard projections that create along the edges of bones)

- squeezed nerve in the neck or shoulder

- broken shoulder or arm bone

- solidified shoulder

- separated shoulder

- injury because of abuse or dreary use

- spinal rope injury

- respiratory failure

How is the reason for shoulder torment analyzed?

Your primary care physician will need to discover the reason for your shoulder torment. They'll demand your clinical history and do a physical assessment.

They'll feel for delicacy and expanding and will likewise evaluate your scope of movement and joint security. Imaging tests, for example, a X-beam or MRI, can create definite photos of your shoulder to help with the conclusion.

Your PCP may likewise pose inquiries to decide the reason. Questions may include:

- Is the agony in one shoulder or both?
- Did this agony start abruptly? Assuming this is the case, what's happening with you?
- Does the agony move to different regions of your body?

- Would you be able to pinpoint the zone of agony?
- Does it hurt when you're not moving?
- Does it hurt more when you move in specific manners?
- Is it a sharp torment or a dull hurt?
- Has the territory of agony been red, hot, or swollen?
- Does the torment keep you conscious around evening time?
- What aggravates it and what improves it?
- Have you needed to restrict your exercises in light of your shoulder torment?

When would it be a good idea for me to look for clinical assistance?

You should contact your PCP on the off chance that you experience fever, failure to move your shoulder, enduring wounding, warmth and delicacy around the joint, or torment that continues past half a month of home treatment.

In the event that your shoulder torment is unexpected and not identified with a physical issue, call 911 right away. It might be an indication of a respiratory failure. Different indications of a coronary episode include:

- inconvenience relaxing
- chest snugness
- wooziness
- extreme perspiring
- genuine annoyance or jaw

Additionally, call 911 or go to a trauma center quickly on the off chance that you harmed your shoulder and are dying, swollen, or you can see uncovered tissue.

What are the treatment alternatives for shoulder torment?

Treatment will rely upon the reason and seriousness of the shoulder torment. Some treatment alternatives incorporate physical or word related treatment, a sling or shoulder immobilizer, or medical procedure.

Your PCP may likewise endorse medicine, for example, nonsteroidal mitigating drugs (NSAIDs) or corticosteroids. Corticosteroids are ground-breaking mitigating drugs that can be taken by mouth or your primary care physician can infuse into your shoulder.

On the off chance that you've had shoulder medical procedure, trail care directions cautiously.

Some minor shoulder torment can be treated at home. Good to beat all 15 to 20 minutes three or four times each day for a few days can help decrease torment. Utilize an ice sack or envelop ice by a towel since putting ice straightforwardly on your skin can cause frostbite and consume the skin.

Resting the shoulder for a few days before getting back to typical action and staying away from any developments that may cause agony can be useful. Cutoff overhead work or exercises.

Other home medicines incorporate utilizing over-the-counter nonsteroidal calming prescriptions to help decrease agony and irritation and compacting the zone with a flexible gauze to diminish expanding.

How might I forestall shoulder torment?

Straightforward shoulder activities can help extend and fortify muscles and rotator sleeve ligaments. A physical specialist or word related advisor can tell you the best way to do them appropriately.

In the event that you've had past shoulder issues, use ice for 15 minutes subsequent to practicing to forestall future wounds.

In the wake of having bursitis or tendinitis, performing basic scope of-movement practices each day can shield you from getting solidified shoulder.

Treating and Managing Shoulder Pain

Sore shoulder cures

This normal joint issue can influence anybody. Shoulder torment may include the ligament, tendons, muscles, nerves, or ligaments. It can likewise incorporate the shoulder bone, neck, arm, and hand.

Early treatment is significant. It can take two months or longer for shoulder agony to recuperate. At-home shoulder torment cures may support recuperation.

Simple cures at home

Treating shoulder torment frequently includes relieving irritation (expanding and redness) and fortifying muscles. Here are a few different ways you can deal with yourself and mitigate shoulder torment.

Mitigating prescription

Nonsteroidal mitigating meds (NSAIDS) help to alleviate agony and lower aggravation. Over-the-counter medications incorporate anti-inflammatory medicine, ibuprofen, and naproxen. Decreasing aggravation is significant in rotator sleeve wounds, tendonitis and joint inflammation, and other shoulder wounds.

Cold pack

Cold packs can help decrease expanding in the shoulder. Cooling likewise assists with desensitizing sharp torment. Apply an ice pack for as long as 20 minutes, up to five times each day. Utilize a solidified gel pack, ice 3D shapes in a plastic sack, or a pack of solidified peas. Enclose the virus pack by a delicate towel. Try not to apply a virus pack legitimately to skin.

Pressure

Wrap the shoulder with a versatile clinical swathe to help diminish expanding and torment. Utilize a chilly pressure wrap or an ordinary ACE gauze. You can likewise get a shoulder wrap from a drug store. Wrap it cozily however not very close. You would prefer not to obstruct blood stream. In the event that your arm or hand starts to feel numb or shivery, or turn blue, release the pressure wrap.

Warmth treatment

Warmth assists with loosening up tense muscles and relieve a hardened shoulder. It can help with muscle torment and joint pain in the shoulder. Utilize a warmed gel pack, warming cushion or a high temp water bottle.

Muscle relaxants

Muscle relaxants may assist treat with tormenting in the event that you have muscle pressure or fits around the shoulder joint. Regular muscle relaxants incorporate cyclobenzaprine, tizanidine, and baclofen. You will require a medicine from your PCP.

Recollect that muscle relaxants cause laziness and shouldn't be taken in case you're driving or working hardware.

Agony prescription

Drugs, for example, acetaminophen and anti-inflammatory medicine can help ease torment. This causes you adapt to the injury and improve rest as you recuperate.

Torment drugs can cause symptoms, for example, stomach upset and acid reflux.

Converse with a specialist in the event that you are taking them for longer than about a month.

You can likewise attempt skin help with discomfort gels and creams, which don't have similar reactions as oral agony prescriptions. Diclofenac is one drug endorsed in two structures by the U.S. Food and Drug Administration for osteoarthritis treatment. It's accessible as 1 percent diclofenac sodium gel and 1.5 percent diclofenac sodium arrangement.

Rest and action alteration

Stop or change the action that may have caused the shoulder torment. It's critical to move the shoulder delicately. This assists with keeping the shoulder muscles solid and adaptable.

Shoulder activities and stretches

Customary activities and stretches can keep your shoulder solid and adaptable. A couple of things to recall before swinging in to works out:

- Stop any activity on the off chance that you have more shoulder torment. It might be too early for you to attempt.
- Watch your structure. Practicing mistakenly can likewise cause or intensify shoulder issues.
- Warm up, even before profound extending. Light shoulder rolls, delicate developments, or even a warm shower are altogether approaching to heat up your muscles before exercise and extending.

Pendulum stretch for scope of movement

- Stand and twist at the midriff.
- Let your arm on the harmed side hang straight down.
- Keep your neck loose.
- Move your arm in a hover up to multiple times.
- Do once or more occasions in a day.

Overhead shoulder stretch

- Sit or remain to do this shoulder stretch.
- Intertwine your fingers before you.
- Bend your elbows and raise your arms over your head. You can likewise put your hands on your head or behind it.
- Gently press your shoulder bones together to move your elbows back.
- Continue for up to 20 reiterations. Rehash 5 to 10 times each day.

When to see a specialist

You'll require treatment alongside home cures in the event that you have a genuine shoulder injury. See your PCP in the event that you have any of the accompanying:

- torment: particularly if the torment doesn't show signs of improvement with rest and drug
- rehash issues: in the event that you have shoulder torment more than once
- solidness: on the off chance that you can't lift and turn your arm typically
- shortcoming: if your shoulder, arm, or hand is more fragile than the healthy side
- isolated or disjoined shoulder: on the off chance that you have a disengagement or in the event that it seems like your shoulder could slide out

Forestalling shoulder torment

The initial step is to rest enough to permit your body to mend and restore from ordinary stressors. Eating a sound, adjusted eating regimen can likewise keep your body energized with the supplements it uses to work.

In case you're encountering a throbbing painfulness, have a go at abstaining from smoking. Smoking can influence blood flow to the shoulder and body. This can slow recuperation.

A shoulder injury can occur with rehash or unexpected developments. It can occur while playing sports, working out, or falling, and during ordinary exercises, for example, going after something on a rack or cultivating. This is almost certain on the off chance that you raise your arms over your head or lift something hefty without bowing the elbows or utilizing your legs to lift the weight.

On the off chance that you have helpless stance or sluggard your shoulders, you might be bound to get shoulder torment.

At the specialist's office

In the event that you have a genuine rotator sleeve tear or a shoulder separation, you may require medical procedure to fix it. Your primary care physician may suggest steroid infusions if the injury doesn't improve or if the torment is extreme. This assists with bringing down irritation.

Shoulder arthroscopy is a key-gap sort of medical procedure. A specialist makes a little gap and uses a minuscule camera to inspect and help fix torn tissue.

Osteoarthritis can cause constant shoulder torment. Pro joint specialists regularly suggest steroid infusions, medical procedure, or shoulder joint substitution medical procedure in intense cases.

Basic causes

Basic conditions that include shoulder torment include:

- joint inflammation
- bursitis
- solidified shoulder
- muscle strain
- rotator sleeve injury
- tendinitis

Diagnosing shoulder torment causes you and your PCP pick the best treatment and home solutions for you.

The Best Exercises for Arthritis in the Shoulders

Joint inflammation in the shoulders

Having joint inflammation can regularly feel like you need a shoulder to incline toward, particularly if it's your shoulder that harms.

Each shoulder contains a joint upheld by muscles, tendons, and ligaments. Joint pain causes irritation in the joints, incorporating those in your shoulder, just as a breakdown of the ligament that pads your bones. This causes the trademark torment and solidness of joint inflammation.

There are more than 100 unique sorts of joint inflammation. The three primary sorts are osteoarthritis (OA), rheumatoid joint pain (RA), and psoriatic joint pain (PsA). Each type grows in an unexpected way, and all require distinctive clinical treatment. In any case, certain exercises can help calm joint inflammation manifestations.

Following are a few hints for practicing when you have joint inflammation in your shoulders.

Cycle through the torment

Cycling is one of the best approaches to practice with joint inflammation shoulder torment. On the off chance that you ride your bicycle outside or utilize a fixed bicycle inside, ensure the handlebars are at a proper level. In the event that they're excessively low, you'll wind up putting more strain on effectively firm shoulder joints.

Attempt a prostrate bicycle without handlebars for indoor cycling. This spots more spotlight on your legs and center. Mixture bikes will in general be the most ideal choices for outside. That is a result of the higher handlebar arrangement and upstanding sitting position.

Exploit rec center participations

Not many individuals have the space or cash to put resources into expand rec center gear. A rec center participation is the ideal other option. At the rec center, exploit the cardio machines. They can push you to:

- condition your body
- advance sound stance
- ease the heat off your shoulder joints

Think about utilizing the accompanying machines:

- circular
- treadmill
- step stepper
- fixed bicycle

"*Push up*" *against shoulder torment*

Pushups are viewed as outstanding amongst other all-around works out. They work muscles in your chest area and center while expanding your metabolic rate. You can at present do pushups with shoulder joint pain, however you'll have to make a few adjustments.

Rather than driving ceaselessly the floor, consider divider pushups. This technique can guarantee better arrangement and less shoulder strain. Play out a couple of reps daily. Possibly increment the term on the off chance that you don't encounter any agony. You shouldn't have torment whenever while doing pushups.

Discover your "om"

Yoga is known for building quality and adaptability. It additionally consolidates breathing activities for refined development. This sort of exercise is viable for shoulder joint pain. It reinforces both the upper and lower body without the high effect of some different exercises.

Talk with your educator about adjusting some yoga positions for your condition. Stay away from represents that will add additional strain to the shoulders or cause any extra shoulder torment. Yet in addition don't restrict practice prospects. In the event that you can do Downward-Facing Dog without torment, at that point it's a decent exercise to do.

Try not to preclude strolling

You may stroll to consume off fat or some steam. However, customary strolling may even assist you with consuming off shoulder torment. This low-sway exercise is best when you stand up tall with your shoulders back.

An everyday walk can improve your state of mind and can hold your weight in line. It might likewise help decline expanding and solidness in your joints.

Tips for lifting loads

Quality preparing assumes a key part in expanding bulk and bone thickness. In the event that you have joint pain in your shoulder, you may accept that you can't lift loads any longer. In any case, that isn't altogether evident.

The key is to zero in on practices that don't need raising loads over your shoulders or create any extra agony. Focus on any agony. The sign your joints are getting more kindled or bothered.

Customary bicep twists, seat presses, paddling, and pectoral chest flies are altogether suitable. The American College of Rheumatology prescribes 8 to 10 reps of every quality preparing exercise, up to three times each week.

Try not to bear the weight alone

Practicing to ease shoulder joint inflammation requires a significant level of responsibility. Having an emotionally supportive network is basic. Welcome your relatives to practice with you, or enroll the assistance of companions for additional inspiration and consolation.

Remember to talk about your activity plans with your primary care physician and physical specialist first. They'll ensure your exercises are sheltered and can give you some additional tips for progress.

While you shouldn't perform practices that expansion your agony, don't altogether abstain from turning out to be either.

Step by step instructions to Identify and Correct a Dislocated Shoulder

Manifestations of a separated shoulder

An unexplained torment in your shoulder can mean numerous things, including separation. At times, distinguishing a disengaged shoulder is as simple as glancing in the mirror. The influenced region might be noticeably deformed with an unexplained bump or lump.

As a rule, however, different manifestations will demonstrate separation. Notwithstanding expanding and extreme agony, a disengaged shoulder can cause muscle fits. These wild developments can exacerbate your torment. The torment may likewise go all over your arm, beginning at your shoulder and climbing toward your neck.

When to look for clinical consideration

In the event that your shoulder has separated from the joint, it's significant that you see your PCP immediately to forestall further agony and injury.

As you hold on to see your PCP, don't move your shoulder or attempt to push it once again into the right spot. On the off chance that you attempt to push the shoulder once more into the joint all alone, you hazard harming your shoulder and joint, just as the nerves, tendons, veins, and muscles here.

Rather, attempt to brace or sling your shoulder set up to shield it from moving until you can see a specialist. What tops off an already good thing help decrease agony and growing. Ice may likewise help control any interior draining or development of liquids around the joint.

How a disengaged shoulder is analyzed

At your arrangement, your primary care physician will get some information about:

- how you harmed your shoulder
- how long your shoulder has been harming
- what different manifestations you've encountered
- on the off chance that this ever occurred previously

Knowing precisely how you disjoined your shoulder — regardless of whether it was from a fall, sport injury, or some other sort of mishap — can enable your PCP to more readily evaluate your physical issue and treat your indications.

Your primary care physician will likewise see how well you can move your shoulder and verify whether you feel any distinction in torment or deadness as you move it. He will check your heartbeat to make sure there is no related injury to a course. Your PCP will likewise evaluate for any nerve injury.

Much of the time, your primary care physician may take a X-beam to improve thought of your physical issue. A X-beam will show any extra injury to the shoulder joint or any messed up bones, which are normal with disengagements.

Treatment choices

After your primary care physician has an away from of your physical issue, your treatment will start. To begin, your PCP will give a shut decrease a shot your shoulder.

Shut decrease

This implies your PCP will push your shoulder once more into your joint. You specialist may give you a mellow soothing or a muscle relaxer heretofore to help decrease any inconvenience. A X-beam will be performed after the decrease to affirm that the shoulder is the best possible position.

When your shoulder is held up once again into your joint, your torment ought to die down.

Immobilization

When your shoulder has been reset, your primary care physician may utilize a brace or sling to shield your shoulder from moving as it mends. Your PCP will prompt you on how long to keep the shoulder stable. Contingent upon your physical issue, it might be anyplace from a couple of days to three weeks.

Drug

As you proceed to recuperate and recover quality in your shoulder, you may require medicine to help with the agony. Your PCP may propose ibuprofen (Motrin) or acetaminophen (Tylenol). You can likewise apply an ice pack to help with the agony and growing.

In the event that your PCP thinks you need something more grounded, they will suggest original effectiveness ibuprofen or acetaminophen, which you can get from a drug specialist. They may likewise recommend hydrocodone or tramadol.

Medical procedure

In extreme cases, careful mediation might be vital. This methodology is a final retreat and is possibly utilized if a shut decrease has fizzled or if there is broad harm to the encompassing veins and muscles. On uncommon events, a disengagement can have a related vascular physical issue, either to a significant vein or course. This can require pressing medical procedure. Medical procedure on the case or other delicate tissues might be fundamental, yet generally sometime in the future.

Recovery

Physical recovery can assist you with recapturing your quality and improve your scope of movement. Recovery by and large incorporates managed or guided exercise at a non-intrusive treatment community. Your PCP will suggest a physical specialist and prompt you on your following stages.

The sort and length of your recovery will rely upon the degree of your physical issue. It could take a couple of arrangements for every week for a month or more.

Your physical specialist may likewise give you practices for you to do at home. There might be sure positions you have to keep away from to forestall another disengagement, or they may suggest certain activities dependent on the sort of separation you had. It's imperative to do them routinely and adhere to any directions the advisor gives.

You shouldn't take an interest in sports or any arduous action until your PCP believes it's protected enough to do as such. Taking part in these exercises before you are cleared by your PCP can harm your shoulder considerably more.

Home consideration

You can ice your shoulder with ice or cold packs to help with the torment and irritation. Apply a virus pack to your shoulder for 15 to 20 minutes one after another each couple of hours for the initial 2 days.

You can likewise give a hot pack a shot the shoulder. The warmth will help loosen up your muscles. You can attempt this strategy for 20 minutes one after another as you feel the need.

Standpoint

It can take somewhere in the range of 12 to about four months to totally recoup from a disengaged shoulder.

Following fourteen days, you ought to have the option to restore most exercises of day by day living. Nonetheless, you ought to follow your doctor's particular proposal.

On the off chance that you will probably re-visitation of sports, planting, or different exercises that incorporate hard work, your primary care physician's direction is much more pivotal. Taking an interest in these exercises too early can additionally harm your shoulder and may keep you from these exercises later on.

By and large, it can take somewhere in the range of about a month and a half to 3 months before you can partake in difficult movement once more. Contingent upon your activity, this may mean getting some much-needed rest work or incidentally moving to another job.

Converse with your PCP about the choices accessible to you. With appropriate consideration, your separated shoulder will mend appropriately and you'll have the option to continue your everyday movement before you know it.

Shoulder Impingement Test: Important Tool for Evaluating Your Shoulder Pain

In the event that you figure you may have shoulder impingement disorder; a specialist may allude you to a physical advisor (PT) who will perform tests to help distinguish precisely where the impingement is found and the best treatment plan.

Regular tests incorporate the Neer, Hawkins-Kennedy, coracoid impingement, and cross-arm impingement tests, alongside a few others. During these evaluations, a PT will request that you move your arms in various ways to check for agony and portability issues.

Studies Trusted Source uphold utilizing a few distinct evaluations to perceive what constraints you're encountering and what triggers the agony.

"Physical specialists don't balance their caps on one test. A large number of tests drives us to an analysis," said Steve Vighetti, an individual of the American Academy of Orthopedic Manual Physical Therapists.

Related to symptomatic imaging

Numerous specialists use X-beams, CT checks, MRI sweeps, and ultrasound testing to explain and affirm the aftereffects of physical assessments.

Studies show that imaging tests are exceptionally viable at pinpointing the exact area of a physical issue. Ultrasound has the upside of being anything but difficult to perform and more affordable than other imaging tests.

In the event that there are tears, or injuries, in the rotator sleeve, imaging tests can show the level of the injury and assist specialists with deciding if a fix is expected to reestablish your capacities.

What precisely is a shoulder impingement?

Shoulder impingement is an excruciating condition. It happens when the ligaments and delicate tissues around your shoulder joint become caught between the head of your upper arm bone (the humerus) and the acromion, a hard projection that expands upward from your scapula (shoulder bone).

At the point when the delicate tissues are pressed, they can become disturbed or even tear, causing you torment and restricting your capacity to move your arm appropriately.

For what reason do you need an exhaustive physical test?

The expression "shoulder impingement disorder" is only the beginning stage to a right determination and treatment plan.

"It's a trick all expression," Vighetti said. "It just reveals to you that a ligament is aggravated. What a decent physical specialist will do is figure out which ligaments and muscles are included."

What are the kinds of impingement tests, and what occurs during each?

Neer test or Neer sign

In the Neer test, the PT remains behind you, pushing down on the head of your shoulder. At that point, they turn your arm internal toward your chest and raise your arm the extent that it will go.

Some studies Trusted Source show that the altered Neer test has an indicative exactness pace of 90.59 percent.

Hawkins-Kennedy test

During the Hawkins-Kennedy test, you're situated while the PT remains next to you. They flex your elbow to a 90-degree point and raise it to bear level. Their arm goes about as a support underneath your elbow while they push down on your wrist to turn your shoulder.

Coracoid impingement test

The coracoid impingement test works this way: The PT remains next to you and raises your arm to bear level with your elbow twisted at a 90-degree point. Supporting your elbow, they push down tenderly on your wrist.

Yocum test

In the Yocum test, you place one hand on your contrary shoulder and raise your elbow without raising your shoulder.

Cross-arm test

In the cross-arm test, you raise your arm to bear level with your elbow flexed at a 90-degree edge. At that point, keeping your arm in a similar plane, you move it over your body at chest level.

The PT may delicately press your arm as you arrive at the end scope of movement.

Jobe's test

During Jobe's test, the PT stands to your side and somewhat behind you. They raise your arm out aside. At that point, they move the arm to the front of your body and request that you keep it raised in that position while they push down on it.

These tests intend to diminish the measure of room between the delicate tissues and bone. The tests can progressively turn out to be more serious as the PT's assessment moves along.

"We'll leave the most agonizing tests for the finish of the appraisal so the shoulder isn't aggravated the entire time," Vighetti said. "On the off chance that you do an excruciating test too soon, at that point the consequences of the apparent multitude of tests will have all the earmarks of being positive."

What are they searching for?

Torment

A test is viewed as certain on the off chance that it inspires a similar torment you've been encountering in your shoulder. The Neer test, Vighetti stated, will regularly get a positive outcome, since it powers the arm into full flexion.

"You're toward the end scope of movement with the Neer test," he said. "Nearly any individual who comes into the center with a shoulder issue will encounter squeezing at the upper finish of that extend."

Area of the torment

During each test, the PT gives close consideration to where your torment happens. This shows which part of your shoulder complex is probably going to be encroached or harmed.

Agony at the rear of the shoulder, for instance, could be an indication of an inside impingement. When advisors realize which muscles are included, they can be more explicit in their medicines.

Muscle work

Regardless of whether you're not encountering torment during a test, the muscles associated with shoulder impingement have a somewhat extraordinary reaction to pressure testing.

"We utilize light, two-finger protection from test explicit movements at the rotator sleeve," Vighetti said. "In the event that somebody objects to the rotator sleeve, even that truly light opposition will inspire indications."

Portability and joint security issues

"Agony is the thing that acquires patients," Vighetti brought up. "In any case, there is a hidden issue causing the agony. In some cases, the issue is identified with joint versatility. The joint is moving excessively or insufficient. In the event that the joint is insecure, the sleeve is pivoting hard to attempt to give dynamic strength."

At the point when muscles work this difficult, issues can emerge — not really on the grounds that the muscles are abused but since they're being utilized erroneously.

Hence, a decent PT takes a gander at the exercises you do to check whether you're moving such that will to injury. Vighetti tapes exercises like hurrying to recognize any disfunction in the development.

The reality

Specialists and PTs utilize demonstrative imaging and physical assessments to distinguish where and how much your shoulder might be harmed.

During the physical test, a PT will take you through a progression of movements to attempt to reproduce the torment you're feeling as you move your arm in various ways. These tests help the PT discover where you're harmed.

The primary objectives of treatment are to diminish your torment, increment your scope of movement, make you more grounded and your joints more steady, and train your muscles to move such that makes future wounds more outlandish.

"It's about training," Vighetti said. "Great physical advisors show patients how to oversee all alone."

Instructions to Identify and Correct a Dislocated Shoulder

Indications of a disjoined shoulder

An unexplained agony in your shoulder can mean numerous things, including separation. At times, recognizing a disengaged shoulder is as simple as glancing in the mirror. The influenced zone might be obviously distorted with an unexplained protuberance or lump.

As a rule, however, different side effects will demonstrate disengagement. Notwithstanding growing and extreme torment, a separated shoulder can cause muscle fits. These wild developments can exacerbate your agony. The agony may likewise go here and there your arm, beginning at your shoulder and climbing toward your neck.

When to look for clinical consideration

On the off chance that your shoulder has separated from the joint, it's significant that you see your primary care physician immediately to forestall further torment and injury.

As you stand by to see your PCP, don't move your shoulder or attempt to push it once again into the right spot. In the event that you attempt to push the shoulder once more into the joint all alone, you hazard harming your shoulder and joint, just as the nerves, tendons, veins, and muscles here.

Rather, attempt to brace or sling your shoulder set up to shield it from moving until you can see a specialist. What tops off an already good thing help lessen torment and growing. Ice may likewise help control any interior draining or development of liquids around the joint.

How a disjoined shoulder is analyzed

At your arrangement, your PCP will get some information about:

- how you harmed your shoulder
- how long your shoulder has been harming

what different side effects you've encountered?

in the event that this ever occurred previously

Knowing precisely how you disengaged your shoulder — regardless of whether it was from a fall, sport injury, or some other sort of mishap — can enable your primary care physician to all the more likely survey your physical issue and treat your indications.

Your PCP will likewise see how well you can move your shoulder and verify whether you feel any distinction in torment or deadness as you move it. He will check your heartbeat to make sure there is no related injury to a vein. Your PCP will likewise evaluate for any nerve injury.

By and large, your primary care physician may take a X-beam to show signs of improvement thought of your physical issue. A X-beam will show any extra injury to the shoulder joint or any wrecked bones, which are normal with disengagements.

4 Shoulder Stretches You Can Do at Work

What causes shoulder torment?

We will in general partner shoulder torment with sports, for example, tennis and baseball, or with the repercussions of moving around our parlor furniture. Few could actually presume that the reason is regularly something as normal and inert as sitting at our work areas.

In any case, notably, gazing at our PC screens for over eight hours daily can enormously affect our shoulders' deltoid, subclavius, and trapezius muscles.

PC work can cause shoulder torment

The American Academy of Orthopedic Surgeons appraises that the regular PC client hits their console up to 200,000 times each day.

Over the long haul, these dreary developments from a moderately fixed situation for quite a long time at a stretch can unleash destruction on your musculoskeletal wellbeing. It can prompt:

- terrible stance

- cerebral pains
- joint agony

The World Health Organization and other driving clinical foundations characterize these kinds of shoulder wounds, frequently in blend with neck and back strain, as musculoskeletal issues.

Exercise can help forestall shoulder torment

Fortunately, Dr. Dustin Tavenner of the Lakeshore Chiropractic and Rehabilitation Center in Chicago as often as possible treats individuals who have shoulder torment related with extended periods of time of sitting.

Tavenner suggests these four simple and snappy shoulders extends that you can accomplish at work to help mitigate shoulder torment.

Work area heavenly attendants

Sitting straight in your seat with impeccable stance, place your arms at shoulder level with a 90-degree twist in your elbows.

Keeping your head and middle fixed, gradually move your arms overhead, arriving at your hands toward the roof. Attempt to keep your arms in accordance with your ears as you climb to the roof and gradually back to the beginning position.

You should feel some pulling in your midback, which assists with loosening up your spine.

Rehash multiple times.

- Shoulder rolls

- Keep your back straight and your jawline took care of.
- Roll your shoulders forward, up, back, and down in a round movement.
- Rehash multiple times, at that point turn around.

Upper trapezius stretches

- Sitting with your back straight, tilt your head sideways toward your shoulder.
- For a bigger stretch, drop your shoulder bone on the contrary side toward the floor.
- Hold for 10 seconds.
- Rehash twice on each side.

Armpit stretches

This stretch will make it appear as though you're attempting to smell your own armpit, so maybe you ought to play out this one when you're certain nobody is looking.

- Sit with your back straight.
- Pivot your head sideways with the goal that your nose is legitimately over your armpit.
- Hold the rear of your head with your hand and use it to delicately push your nose nearer to your armpit. Try not to push to the point of uneasiness.
- Hold for 10 seconds.
- Rehash twice on each side.

Continue with control

Notwithstanding these stretches, "dynamic" sitting can keep your body moving and forestall the agony that outcomes from being inactive. For instance, recline in your seat infrequently, turn your seat from side to side, and stay standing for a couple of seconds in any event once consistently.

As usual, be cautious while adding another activity to your day by day schedule. Should you keep on encountering agony or uneasiness, converse with your PCP.

The most effective method to Prevent Shoulder Injuries

In regular day to day existence, your shoulder gets a genuine exercise. It moves pretty much every time you do. You use it for lifting, coming to, or in any event, tossing a ball. You can get something high or take something out the ground.

You can do every one of these things on the grounds that a sound shoulder has an incredible scope of movement, and that is something worth being thankful for. However, all that development implies there are more ways for you to get injured. The shoulder is the body's most harmed joint.

The most widely recognized issues originate from rehashing a similar development again and again, and from an excessive amount of arm movement over your head (like composition or hanging shades).

In any case, your shoulder can get injured in different manners as well:

Age. Characteristic mileage that accompanies age can harm your shoulder.

Osteoarthritis. The ligament (extreme rubbery cushioning) that secures your joints wears out.

Rotator sleeve harm. The rotator sleeve is a gathering of muscles and ligaments that keeps your shoulder together.

Bursitis. The liquid filled cushions that pad your joints get swollen.

Separation. Your upper arm bone emerges from the shoulder (it ordinarily fits like an attachment). This can hurt a ton.

Solidified shoulder. The case of connective tissue that holds your shoulder together thickens and fixes around the joint, limiting its development.

Avoidance

Fortunately, shoulder issues frequently can be fixed without medical procedure. In any case, it's ideal to evade the issue in any case. Here are a few different ways to do that.

Tune in to your body. On the off chance that your shoulder gets sore after any movement, don't disregard it. On the off chance that the torment is not kidding and doesn't disappear, see your PCP. There's no compelling reason to endure it. You very well might compound the situation.

Remain fit as a fiddle. Keep your body fit as a fiddle with standard exercise and a sound eating routine. It's a method to remain well and it can assist you with staying away from injury.

Exercise the correct way. Warm up before you work out. Start gradually on the off chance that you haven't done a game or a movement in some time. Figure out how to lift loads the correct way. Try not to lift excessively.

Watch out grinding away. Ensure you don't harm your shoulder at work.

Utilize great stance when you sit or stand.

Adhere to the principles for safe lifting. Keep your back straight and utilize your legs.

Enjoy a reprieve for two or three minutes consistently. Move around and stretch.

On the off chance that you work at a work area, ensure your work station is set up so you can serenely utilize your PC.

Try not to strain to arrive at what you need. Utilize a stage stool in the event that you need to arrive at high places. Put the things you use in drawers or on lower racks.

Recuperation

In the event that you do hurt your shoulder, these things should assist you with feeling much improved:

Rest and ice are vital. Apply ice like clockwork.

Inquire as to whether you can assume control over-the-counter torment relievers like headache medicine, ibuprofen, or naproxen.

In the event that your primary care physician recommends exercise-based recuperation, ensure you do it.

Try not to wear a sling. You need to keep your arm allowed to move. Simply don't try too hard.

Tips to Prevent Shoulder Pain

There's nothing more baffling for a competitor than sitting harmed uninvolved watching others contend. In spite of the fact that there's nobody secure approach to prevent shoulder torment from happening, there are a few hints that may help keep it from beginning or deteriorating.

1. Rest. In the event that you notice shoulder torment during specific exercises, state while tossing a baseball or swimming, stop that action for a while and locate an elective exercise, for example, riding a fixed bicycle. Doing so can give your shoulder some an ideal opportunity to rest and mend, while keeping up your cardiovascular wellness.

Simultaneously, don't kill all shoulder development. This is on the grounds that you would prefer not to build up a hardened shoulder from rare use. Consider doing some gentle stretches to keep your arm moving.

2. **Change your dozing position.** In the event that you notice torment in your correct shoulder, don't rest on your correct side. Give dozing a shot your left side or back. In the event that dozing on your back disturbs your shoulder, take a stab at propping your arm up with a cushion.

3. **Warm up.** Practicing cold muscles is never a smart thought. Before rehearsing your volleyball serve or baseball throw, warm up your body with gentle exercise. For instance, begin strolling for a couple of moments and bit by bit develop to a run. Doing so raises your pulse and internal heat level and actuates the synovial liquid (grease) in your joints.1 as

such, a mellow warm up prepares your body for the serious exercise that follows.

4. **Develop your perseverance.** It's a smart thought to build your continuance after some time. On the off chance that it's been half a month or months since you've hit the tennis court, think about playing for a brief timeframe—possibly only 20 minutes to begin—and develop to a more extended time of playing time. Try not to fall into the snare of doing an excess of too early, particularly when your body isn't utilized to it.

5. **Increment your shoulder quality.** Fortifying your shoulder muscles can help offer help and adjustment to your shoulder joint. This, thus, may forestall difficult wounds like a shoulder disengagement, which is the point at

which the wad of your shoulder emerges from its attachment.

Address your PCP before beginning a fortifying project. They can propose activities to perform or may suggest working with a physical specialist.

6. **Broadly educate.** A few games are especially burdening on the shoulder because of dull, overhead developments. So, you may need consider broadly educating. In case you're a swimmer, for instance, substitute a portion of your swimming exercises with a running or biking exercise to lessen the weight on your shoulder, while as yet remaining truly fit.

Then again, in case you're a painter or development laborer—two occupations usually connected with dreary, overhead developments—converse with your chief and inquire as to whether there are other non-redundant errands you can take on.

Most importantly, tune in to your body and be proactive. You may need to make a few acclimations to exercise or every day schedule to help forestall further harm not far off. It might likewise merit getting your PCP's info, regardless of whether you think you have a minor physical issue. Getting wounds or distress early may help keep you in the game and forestall difficult wounds not far off.

5 Tips for Preventing Shoulder Injuries

Not many things are additionally irritating for a competitor or dynamic individual than being sidelined by a shoulder injury. Indeed, even ordinary exercises become a battle when your shoulder harms, and however there's no secure method to forestall agony or wounds, there are a few stages you can take to dodge a physical issue or shield it from deteriorating.

Continuously warm up

Practicing cold muscles is quite often a catastrophe waiting to happen. Shoulder extends and even a short cardio meeting gets your pulse up and actuates the synovial liquid which greases up your joints. A decent warm-up is modest protection against a physical issue that can endure forever.

Increment shoulder quality

Lifting and practicing utilizing appropriate structure to fortify your shoulder can help balance out the joint, assisting with forestalling agonizing separation wounds. Continuously address a specialist before starting a fortifying project. They can help figure out which activities are best for you, or they may suggest working with a physical advisor.

Broadly educate

Particularly for competitors who invest a ton of energy doing overhead movements or even individuals whose positions expect them to work overhead a ton, broadly educating can be an incredible method to dodge injury while keeping up your physical wellness. For instance, in case you're a swimmer, have a go at exchanging a couple of swimming exercises for running or biking to diminish weight on your shoulder.

Rest

Like some other muscle bunch in the body, your shoulder needs an ideal opportunity to rest and recuperate. On the off chance that you notice torment while doing a specific action like tossing a ball or lifting loads, locate an elective exercise to take the heap off the harmed zone. Resting your shoulder doesn't mean surrendering all shoulder development, notwithstanding. Doing so can bring about a hardened shoulder from absence of utilization. Indeed, even mellow stretches can help keep your shoulder moving while it recoups.

Change your resting position

In case you're somebody who dozes on their side, abstain from lying on your harmed shoulder around evening time. Give dozing a shot your opposite side or on your back. On the off chance that you rest on your back and it aggravates your shoulder, propping up your arm with a cushion can help.

The most significant activity is consistently tune in to what your body is letting you know. It isn't unexpected to cause acclimations to your exercises or every day schedule to assist with forestalling lasting harm not far off. Regardless of whether you support only a minor injury, it is ideal to talk with a doctor for their info.

www.ingramcontent.com/pod-product-compliance
Lightning Source LLC
Chambersburg PA
CBHW070823240726
48654CB00007B/451